a little handbook about

topical CBD

A REVOLUTIONARY INGREDIENT
FOR THE SKIN CARE WORLD

kayla fioravanti

Selah Press
PUBLISHING

A Little Handbook about Topical CBD: A Revolutionary Ingredient for the Skincare World

By Kayla Fioravanti, Cosmetic Formulator and Certified Aromatherapist

Editing: Kim Aldrich
Cover Design: Haleigh Doyle

Copyright © 2018 Kayla Fioravanti

ISBN-13: 978-0-578-42183-4
Printed in the United States of America, Published by Selah Press

Notice of Liability: The author has made every effort possible to check and ensure the accuracy of the information and recipes presented in this book. However, the information herein is sold without warranty, either expressed or implied. The author, publisher nor any dealer or distributor of this book will be held liable for any damages caused either directly or indirectly by the instructions, recipes or information contained in this book.

Disclaimer: Information in this book is NOT intended as medical advice, nor for use as diagnosis or treatment of a health problem, nor as a substitute for consulting a licensed medical professional. The contents and information in this book are for informational use only and are not intended to be a substitute for professional medical advice, diagnosis, or treatment. Always seek the advice of your physician or other qualified health provider for medical conditions. Never disregard professional medical advice or delay in seeking it because of something you read in this book or any resource.

To Keegan, who changed my life just by becoming. And inspired my journey into the natural industry decades ago, and even more recently into the world of hemp CBD.

Contents

Introduction

Honestly, I was skeptical about the benefits of hemp CBD as a topical ingredient. And, well, if I'm totally honest, I was inclined to believe that hemp CBD was just another fad in the natural industry. My son Keegan kept telling me to try it. And since I've been in the natural industry for over twenty years, I just assumed it was another product that had some value, but could not possibly be nature's wonder drug like everyone was saying. I wouldn't say I'm a pessimist when it comes to new natural products, but I am someone who wants to see the science—more of a questioner would describe me.

My son is persistent, so I started digging. I saw that a chemist that I've known and trusted for nearly twenty years was doing some testing for a lab in the hemp CBD industry. I figured if I was going to start anywhere, I'd start looking in the direction that someone I trusted was working. So I ordered some samples of full spectrum hemp CBD oil for internal use.

I didn't have time to do any research before my samples arrived, so I just blindly followed the directions on the bottle, which is an abnormality for me. I thought that maybe the hemp CBD might help with the chronic joint pain that had plagued me since I was 16 years old. I had only recently discovered that the pain was a symptom of Ehler's Danlos Syndrome, a genetic connective tissue disorder.

After a day, I discovered that I didn't need to take the anti-inflammatories that had become part of my daily routine. That seemed promising. The next day I felt even better. And on the third day, the symptoms that were about to force me to have a hysterectomy had completely resolved.

Wait! What? I had tried every option medicine had to offer to resolve those symptoms—aromatherapy, herbs, diet, exercise, and a year of prayers, with absolutely no relief. I had not for a moment thought that three days of taking hemp CBD would help me avoid the dreaded hysterectomy I had finally resolved myself to accepting as inevitable.

I called Keegan and told him I was sold out on hemp CBD and ready to jump into the industry head first. I dove deep into the research to understand why hemp CBD actually *was* nature's amazing wonder drug. And despite my own amazing healing, I was still skeptical about hemp CBD as a topical product. I devoured everything I could find on hemp CBD, but found very little that explained why hemp CBD could or would work topically. When I couldn't find answers, I asked on Facebook. Most people said they had no idea how or why it worked topically, but that it did. One person said that the skin has CB1 and CB2 receptors. That bit of information changed my Google searching habits, which led to finding research studies on topical hemp CBD and tons of studies that explained the science. So I dove deep into the research papers and came back out with the information I needed to become a believer.

As a cosmetic formulator, certified aromatherapist, approved educator, and someone who loves explaining science in plain English, I realized my research had revealed an information gap that I could help fill. That "aha" moment led to the book you are reading, and to countless talks being given to present the wonders of hemp CBD as a topical product. I also discovered that many people who were selling topical products were not fully aware of the U.S. Food & Drug Administration (FDA) regulation for cosmetics, which hemp CBD topical products fall directly under. And so the final chapter of this book will address that topic for both laymen and brands alike.

One of the nagging questions that also made me drag my feet on the whole idea of hemp CBD was my own misconception that hemp was so closely related to marijuana that there could be safety concerns. I've been sober since 1992. I did not want to expose myself to anything that could jeopardize my sobriety or anyone else's. I am thrilled to tell you that hemp CBD is completely safe, and I will address that concern in greater detail in the first and second chapters. I am all too aware of my own addictive tendencies and want to be sensitive to others like me.

Chapter 1
The Safety of Hemp CBD

I can personally attest to hemp CBD being non-addictive, but honestly you deserve more. In December 2017 the World Health Organization's Expert Committee on Drug Dependence came out with a statement declaring that cannabidiol (CBD) is not an addictive chemical and poses no threat to public health. The World Health Organization (WHO) also suggested that there is no scientific basis for prohibiting cannabidiol.

The report declared that not only is CBD not addictive, it also shows promising potential for addicts: "Another possible therapeutic application which has been investigated is the use of CBD to treat drug addiction. A recent systematic review concluded that there were a limited number of preclinical studies which suggest that CBD may have therapeutic properties on opioid, cocaine, and psychostimulant addiction, and some preliminary data suggest that it may be beneficial in cannabis and tobacco addiction in humans"[1] (World Health Organization Expert Committee on Drug Dependence 2017).

Some worry that there hasn't been enough research into the safety of hemp CBD. However, I found countless studies *and* studies of studies. An example of thorough research was done by Mateus Machado Bergamashci who completed a comprehensive survey of the safety and side effects of CBD using reports retrieved from *Web of Science, Scielo and Medline*. His research, "Safety and Side Effects of Cannabidiol, a Cannabis sativa Constituent," was published in *Current Drug Safety*. Bergamashci found that CBD is safe for humans and animals[2] (Bergamaschi et al 2011).

In 2011 Iffland Kerstin and Grotenhermen Franjo from the German research center nova-Institut set out to expand on

Bergamaschci's findings with a new comprehensive study, "An Update on Safety and Side Effects of Cannabidiol: A Review of Clinical Data and Relevant Animal Studies." Kerstin and Franjo's studies found that CBD had no adverse effect on blood pressure, heart rate, body temperature, glucose levels, pH, pressure exerted by carbon dioxide or oxygen, hematocrits, gastrointestinal transit, emesis, rectal temperature, potassium and sodium levels, and no reparatory depression or cardiovascular complications. The study also found that even chronic use of CBD in humans caused no neurological, psychiatric, or clinical adverse effects. In even more positive news, the new study found CBD is potentially beneficial in the treatment of heroin addiction, reducing seizures, managing psychosis, inhibiting cancer, and reducing anxiety. They also found that cannabinoid has immunomodulatory and neuroprotective properties[3] (Kerstin Iffland and Franjo Grotenhermen 2017). This is of no surprise, since the American government obtained a patent in 1998 for cannabinoids as antioxidants and neuroprotectants.[4]

Iffland and Grotenhermen also found that hemp CBD has a better side effect profile for the treatment of epilepsy and psychotic disorders, which they believed could improve the compliance and adherence to treatment[5] (Kerstin Iffland and Franjo Grotenhermen 2017). Anyone who has ever suffered through the side effects of any over-the-counter or prescription drug knows exactly how important this finding is for hemp CBD as an alternative therapy for multiple diseases and disorders.

Iffland and Grotenhermen went on to state that, "At lower doses, it [CBD] has physiological effects that promote and maintain health, including antioxidative, anti-inflammatory, and neuroprotection effects. For instance, CBD is more effective than vitamin C and E as a neuroprotective antioxidant and can ameliorate skin conditions such as acne"[6] (Kerstin Iffland and Franjo Grotenhermen 2017).

Chapter 2
Let's Talk Hemp

Both hemp and marijuana come from the same species of plant *Cannabis Sativa L.*, but that is where the similarities end. Hemp is cultivated differently and has completely different functions and applications. Hemp is said to have 25,000 uses. Marijuana has 2 uses—medical and recreational use.

The hemp plant contains a high level of cannabidiol (CBD) and only trace amounts of THC (regulated to 0.3%), while the marijuana plant has the opposite with a 5-30% THC content. THC is the psychoactive constituent of the *Cannibas* plant. Attempting to get high by smoking hemp would be a futile effort. Ministry of Hemp puts it this way, "Your lungs will fail before your brain attains any high from smoking industrial hemp"[1] (Ministry of Hemp 2018).

The hemp plant is the most misunderstood plant. David P. West Ph.D. captured it perfectly when he wrote, "Surely no member of the vegetable kingdom has ever been more misunderstood than hemp. For too many years, emotion—not reason—has guided our policy toward this crop. And nowhere have emotions run hotter than in the debate over the distinction between industrial hemp and marijuana"[2] (David P. West, Ph.D.).

To break it down, hemp and marijuana are different varietals of the plant species *Cannabis*. One could say they are relatives, but scientifically polar opposites. By the legal definition, hemp contains a trace level of THC and a high level of CBD while marijuana has low CBD and high THC. You can get high on marijuana, and you can't get high on hemp. Period.

Imagine for a moment that the poppy seed was as misunderstood as hemp. There are dozens of varieties of poppy flowers. The *Papaver somniferum* includes the variety of poppies known as the red scarlet, which produces opiates. The non-opium varieties of *Papaver somniferum* are completely legal to grow in your back yard. This despite the fact that the trace opiate level in the poppy seeds you buy for baking at the grocery store is actually higher than the trace THC level in hemp. Imagine if all poppy flowers had been banned because of the red scarlet variety. *There would be no lemon poppy seed muffins!*

"The core agricultural differences between medical cannabis and hemp are largely in their genetic parentage and cultivation environment"[3] (Leaf Science 2014). Hemp and marijuana are scientifically divergent and are cultivated in different ways. Hemp has completely different functions and applications than marijuana. For industrial hemp the seeds, hurd, and fiber are harvested. For marijuana the flowering tops of the female plant, which are the source of Tetrahydrocannabinol (THC), are harvested. Hemp is an agricultural crop often referred to as industrial hemp. Marijuana is a horticultural crop. Every part of the hemp plant has a use and potential market.

The oilseed of hemp is used in the cosmetic, soap, nutritional supplement, and food industries. On multiple occasions I have had people tell me that they took hemp oil and it didn't help. When I asked further questions, I discovered that it was hemp seed oil that they were actually taking or rubbing on their body. Hemp seed oil and hemp CBD oil are two very different things. Hemp seed oil is lovely for a salad, but not quite the same thing at all.

Hemp Seed Oil is a rich source of essential omega-3 and omega-6 fatty acids, gamma-linolenic acid, and proteins. It contains less than 10% saturated fats, and 70-80% polyunsaturated fatty acids. It is full of great stuff! Hemp seed oil does have a short shelf life and can quickly go rancid, which is an important reason not to use hemp seed oil to deliver hemp CBD oil.

When you buy hemp seed oil, it is recommended that you keep it in a refrigerator and make sure it is not exposed to light. It is sensitive to temperature fluctuation, so be sure to put it in the back of your fridge and not in the door. Hemp seed oil has many uses in the cosmetic and culinary industries. An unopened bottle of hemp seed oil that is *properly stored* can last as long as 12-14 months. However, once a bottle of hemp seed oil has been opened, it is recommended that it be consumed within 3-6 months.

The hemp plant has even more uses. The fiber and cellulose from hemp stalks are used in the textile, fuel and building industries. Hemp seed oil also has many household, industrial, and technical uses. Hemp oilseed meal is used in animal feed and protein flours and powders. The hulled hemp seed is used in the food industry. The hemp stalk contains blast fibers and inner core. Blast fibers are one of the strongest plant fibers, which makes them a durable fiber for apparel, luggage, footwear and other textiles. Hemp blast fibers are used in the production of biocomposites for household products, insulation, paper, packaging, flooring, hempcrete, mulch, and so forth, and can be used to replace plastics, fiberglass and wood. The hemp inner core of the stalk is used for animal bedding, as a chemical absorbent that can be used after environmental spills, and can be used in farming and gardening. The whole hemp stalk can be used for biomass fuel. Hemp is the ultimate "green" product because it is renewable. Many products made with it are biodegradable and can be used to replace our dependence on non-renewable resources. The annual crop is great for farmers as a low-impact crop. Erik Rothenberg wrote, "These renewable resources will transition our major industries away from depending on non-renewable, fast-disappearing resource bases to being driven and supported on a sustainable economic basis by the annual agri-industrial produce of the Earth's fertile fields"[4] (Erik Rothenberg 2001).

Hemp CBD Oil

Hemp CBD Oil is very different from hemp seed oil. The acronym CBD comes from the word cannabidiol, which is unique to the *Cannabis* plant. Cannabidiol interacts with the endocannabinoid system (ECS), which I will explain in great detail in the next chapter.

Cannabinoids were first isolated by Roger Adams in 1940[5] (Jeanette Jacknin 2016).

You might be wondering about the shelf life of hemp CBD oil, since I mentioned the shelf life of hemp seed oil. The shelf life and stability of a given brand of hemp CBD oil depends heavily on the oil chosen as a carrier. At my company, Ology Essentials, we have chosen Fractionated Coconut Oil because of its super powers as carrier oil. Fractionated Coconut Oil has an indefinite shelf life and a palatable flavor profile that can be described as tasteless and odorless. Fractionated Coconut Oil is a great source of medium-chain triglycerides (MCT), which are used by the body as a quick source of energy. Many health plans actually recommend adding fractionated coconut oil to your diet. *Now are all MCT created the same?* No. Some come from palm oil, which is a great source of MCT but is not a sustainable ingredient. According to Say No to Palm Oil, "The [palm] industry is linked to major issues such as deforestation, habitat degradation, climate change, animal cruelty and indigenous rights abuses in the countries where it is produced, as the land and forests must be cleared for the development of the oil palm plantations"[6] (Say Not to Palm Oil 2018).

Hemp CBD is often sold in three different forms. You will find references to full spectrum, broad spectrum, and isolate. These are important distinctions. Why? One reason is that you rarely want to hear the words, "You're fired" from your employer. So let's talk THC to make sure you make the right buying decisions when it comes to hemp CBD. Hemp CBD by legal definition can contain 0.3% or less THC as measured in the dried flowering portion of the plant. Drug tests for marijuana are pass/fail for the presence of THC. Since hemp CBD does contain 0.3% or less of THC, you can fail a drug test. In a 2018 story that hit the news in Tennessee, a woman took a drug test for a job promotion. Instead of being promoted, she was fired[7] (WSMV News 2018).

If drug screening is part of your job requirements, you should be using a THC-free version of hemp CBD. When shopping for hemp

CBD, if the packaging says "full spectrum" that means the product does contain 0.3% or less of THC. If the product says, "broad spectrum" that means the cannabinoids of THC, THCV, and THCa have been removed, while leaving in the cannabinoids of CBD, CBN, CBDV, CBG, CBC, and CBN. If the product says, "isolate" that means the product was made from a single molecule 99%+ pure CBD without any other cannabinoids, terpenes, plant material, oil, or chlorophyll.

What do you do if the product doesn't disclose whether it is THC-free or full spectrum? I suggest picking up another brand. This is basic information that should be fully disclosed.

Which version works better? The short answer is the one you can take! If having THC in a product makes it impossible for you to take hemp CBD, then the obvious choice is to choose an isolate or broad spectrum hemp CBD. You can't get the healing effect of Hemp CBD if you can't actually take it for one reason or another. Sometimes that comes down to the THC, and other times it comes down to price. Products made with isolates are less expensive.

In theory, full spectrum has an entourage effect. Dr. Robert Pappas explains, "The entourage effect in the cannabis world usually refers to the enhanced effectiveness of the cannabinoids offered by the inclusion of the native terpenes of the plant. Some will also state it to more generally refer to the greater effectiveness of using the whole plant extract as opposed to just a single isolated cannabinoid"[8] (Dr. Robert Pappas 2018).

Chapter 3
Cannabidiol & the Endocannabinoid System

Generally we are taught about just a handful of the systems of the human body. Most people are not aware there is also the endocannabinoid system. Cannabidiol (CBD) interacts with the endocannabinoid system (ECS), which is made up of millions of cannabinoid receptor sites, known as CB1 and CB2. CB1 receptors are mostly found in the brain, connective tissue, central nervous system, organs, gonads, and glands. The CB2 receptors are mostly found in the immune system, and can also be present in the liver, heart, kidneys, spleen, bones, blood vessels, lymph cells, reproductive organs, and the endocrine glands.

The human body always seeks to maintain homeostasis, or more easily stated, to balance bodily functions. The endocannabinoid system maintains equilibrium in the body by seeking to correct anything that gets out of balance, including mood, sleep, hormones, fertility, memory, energy, anxiety, immune response, appetite, pain, and more. Dr. Dustin Sulak states, "In each tissue, the endocannabinoid system performs different tasks, but the goal is always the same: homeostasis, the maintenance of a stable internal environment despite fluctuations in the external environment"[1] (Dustin Sulak, D.O. 2016).

What is so important about homeostasis? Health, survival, wellness. "Homeostasis, from the Greek words for 'same' and 'steady,' refers to any process that living things use to actively maintain fairly stable conditions necessary for survival"[2] (Emeritus Professor Kelvin Rodolfo).

Even though the human body produces cannabinoid, it is possible to have cannabinoid deficiency. In a study on PubMed, E.B. Russo explains, "Migraine, fibromyalgia, IBS and related conditions display common clinical, biochemical and pathophysiological patterns that suggest an underlying clinical endocannabinoid deficiency that may be suitably treated with cannabinoid medicines"[3] (Russo 2004).

The average American diet has not contained cannabinoids, until recently with the rise of Hemp CBD oil, which contains cannabidiol as well as over 85 other cannabinoids. The plant genus *Cannabis* is the only source, outside the human body, that produces cannabinoids.

Cannabinoids are divided into two groups:

1. Endocannabinoids, which are produced naturally by the endocannabinoid system.

2. Phyto-cannabinoids, which are found in the *Cannabis* plant.

When talking about hemp CBD, we are referring to phyto-cannabinoids.

Systems of the Body

To better understand the job of the endocannabinoid system, it is important to quickly review the other body systems that it helps regulate.

Cardiovascular System: includes the heart, blood, and vessels (veins, arteries and capillaries). A few common ailments of the cardiovascular system include: atherosclerosis (hardening of the arteries caused by high fat diets), heart attack, stroke, hypertension, and heart failure.

Respiratory System: includes the nose, trachea, lungs, and rib muscles. A few common ailments of the respiratory system include: cold, tonsillitis, laryngitis, bronchitis, asthma, emphysema, lung cancer, and tuberculosis.

Skeletal System: includes bones and joints. A few common ailments of the skeletal system include: osteoporosis, leukemia, scoliosis, and Ehler's Danlos syndrome.

Urinary System: includes the bladder, kidneys, ureters, and the urethra. A few common ailments of the urinary system include: kidney stones, bladder infection, and incontinence.

Muscular System: includes the muscles and tendons. A few common ailments of the muscular system include: strain, sprain, spasms, tears, tendinitis, fibromyalgia, muscular dystrophy, Ehler's Danlos syndrome, and tetanus.

Endocrine System: includes glands and hormones. A few common ailments of the endocrine system include: thyroid cancer, metabolic disorders, hypothyroidism, Hashimotos, and Grave's disease.

Digestive System: includes the mouth, esophagus, stomach, intestines, throat, liver, gall bladder, pancreas, rectum, and anus. A few common ailments of the digestive system include: abdominal pain, bloating, constipation, heartburn, diarrhea, nausea, and vomiting.

Nervous System: includes the brain, spinal cord, and nerves. A few common ailments of the nervous system include: Alzheimer's disease, epilepsy, carpal tunnel syndrome, cerebral palsy, multiple sclerosis, encephalitis, and Parkinson's disease.

Lymphatic System: includes the lymph, lymph nodes, lymphatic vessels, lymphatic capillaries, and the spleen. A few common ailments of the lymphatic system include: swollen lymph nodes, lymphadenophathy, cancers, and Hodgkin's disease.

Integumentary System: includes the epidermis, dermis, hydro-dermis, hair follicles, sweat pores, sweat glands, oil glands, and sensory receptors. A few common ailments of the integumentary system include: eczema, psoriasis, skin cancer, dermatitis, hives, and Ehler's Danlos syndrome.

Olfactory System: includes specialized sensory cells known as olfactory sensory neurons, which send messages to your brain. Every olfactory neuron contains one odor receptor. A few common ailments of the olfactory system include: anosmia, dysosmia, hyperosmia, and hyposmia.

Immune System: includes a network of cells, tissues, and organs that work together to respond to "foreign" invaders such as bacteria, parasites, viruses, and fungi. White blood cells (leukocytes) circulate in the body between organs and lymph nodes via lymphatic vessels and blood vessels. Leukocytes can be either *phagocytes,* which are cells that chew up invading organisms, or *lymphocytes,* which are cells that allow the body to recall and recognize previous "foreign" invaders. This helps the body to destroy returning invaders. A few common ailments of the immune system include: autoimmune diseases (e.g. Type 1 diabetes, rheumatoid arthritis, and lupus), immunodeficiency, allergies, AIDS, HIV, and asthma.

Reproductive System: includes internal and external organs involved in procreation. The male reproductive system includes the testes and the penis. The female reproductive system can be divided into internal and external structures. The external includes: the clitoris, labia minora, labia majora, and Bartholin's glands. The internal includes: vagina, uterus, ovaries, cervix, and fallopian tubes. A few examples of common ailments of the reproductive system include: endometriosis, cancers (prostate, breast, ovarian, uterine, and testicular), infertility, and fibroids.

Geeking Out Further on Cannabidiol
The National Institute of Health has defined cannabidiol. Even a science geek can benefit from a few plain English translations added. Everything in parenthesis below has been added to the text as definitions and not part of the original definition.

"Cannabidiol is a phytocannabinoid (naturally occurring

cannabinoid) from *Cannabis* species, which is devoid (not possessing) of psychoactive (affecting the mind) activity, with analgesic (acting to relieve pain), anti-inflammatory, antineoplastic (acting to prevent, inhibit or halt the development of a neoplasm/tumor) and chemopreventive (use of a drug to slow or prevent the development of cancer) activities. Upon administration, cannabidiol [CBD] exerts its anti-proliferative (to not grow or multiply by rapidly producing new tissue, parts, cells, or offspring), anti-angiogenic (a naturally occurring substance, drug, or other compound that can destroy or interfere with the fine network of blood vessels needed by tumors to grow and metastasize) and pro-apoptotic (promoting or causing cell self-destruction, a normal physiological process eliminating DNA-damaged, superfluous, or unwanted cells) activity through various mechanisms, which likely do not involve signaling by cannabinoid receptor 1 [CB1] (cannabinoid receptors are primarily located on nerve cells in the brain, spinal cord, but they are also found in some peripheral organs and tissues such as the spleen, white blood cells, endocrine gland, and parts of the reproductive, gastrointestinal and urinary tracts), CB2 (immune cells mainly found on white blood cells, in the tonsils and in the spleen), or vanilloid receptor 1 [TRPV1] (The validation of TRPV1 receptor as a key therapeutic target for pain management has thrust intensive drug discovery programs aimed at developing orally active antagonists of the receptor protein). CBD stimulates endoplasmic reticulum (ER) stress (malfunction of the ER stress response caused by aging, genetic mutations, or environmental factors can result in various diseases such as diabetes, inflammation, and neurodegenerative disorders including Alzheimer's disease, Parkinson's disease, and bipolar disorder, which are collectively known as 'conformational diseases) and inhibits AKT/mTOR signaling (intracellular signaling pathway important in regulating the cell cycle), thereby activating autophagy (a self-degradative process that is important for balancing sources of energy) and promoting apoptosis (a genetically directed process of cell self-destruction that is marked by the fragmentation of nuclear DNA). In addition, CBD enhances the generation of reactive oxygen species [ROS] (type of unstable molecule that contains oxygen and that easily reacts with other molecules in a cell), which further enhances apoptosis (a genetically directed process of cell self-destruction that is marked by the fragmentation of nuclear DNA). This agent also upregulates (the process of increasing the response to a stimulus) the expression of intercellular adhesion molecule 1 [ICAM-1] (part of the immunoglobulin superfamily and are important in inflammation, immune responses and in intracellular signalling events) and tissue inhibitor of matrix metalloproteinases-1 [TIMP1] (key regulators of the metalloproteinases that degrade the extracellular matrix and shed cell surface molecules) and decreases the expression of inhibitor of DNA binding 1 [ID-1] (overexpression is associated with cancers). This inhibits cancer cell invasiveness (tending to invade healthy tissue) and metastasis (cancer cells break away from the original [primary] tumor, travel through the blood or lymph system, and form a new tumor in other organs or tissues of the body). CBD may also activate the transient receptor potential vanilloid type 2 [TRPV2] (expressed in immune cells), which may increase the uptake of various cytotoxic agents (a substance that kills cells, including cancer cells which may stop cancer cells from dividing and growing and may cause tumors to shrink in size) in cancer cells. The analgesic (acting to relieve pain) effect of CBD is mediated through the binding of this agent to and activation of CB1"[4] (U.S. National Institute of Health).

Chapter 4
Going Beyond Skin Deep

Skin is the largest organ in the body and there are cannabinoid receptor sites located throughout the skin. In fact, the skin contains countless cannabinoid receptors—even the sebaceous glands and hair follicles contain endocannabinoid receptors.

Because cannabinoid receptors are located all throughout the skin, CBD has the capability of interacting with endocannabinoid receptors to encourage not only homeostasis, but also healing. A 2005 study found that the distribution of CB1 and CB2 receptors were observed in cutaneous nerve fiber bundles, mast cells, macrophages, epidermal keratinocytes, and the epithelial cells of hair follicles, sebocytes and eccrine sweat glands. Cannabinoid receptors have even been found in the smallest nerve fibers that control hair follicles[1] (Stånder et al 2005).

A 2003 study showed that keratinocytes (epidermal cells that produce keratin) are part of the endocannabinoid system. The study concluded that, "we report evidence that human keratinocytes have a functional 'endocannabinoid system,' which may sustain the peripheral actions of AEA at the skin level. Our findings give a biochemical foundation for the effects of AEA on epidermal cells, especially in relation to pain sensation, response to UV irradiation, cell proliferation, and tumor growth. In this context, the finding that human keratinocytes partake in the peripheral endocannabinoid system and that AEA can inhibit epidermal differentiation opens new perspectives in the understanding of skin development and in the treatment of human skin diseases where cell hyperproliferation takes place"[2] (Maccarrone et al 2003).

Another reason Hemp CBD is the next best thing in skincare and personal care products is that CBD binds to TRPV-1 receptors found in the skin, which are responsible for the sensations of heat, itch, and pain, making it an excellent ingredient for psoriasis, eczema, cystic acne, and more[3] (Tamás Bíró et al 2009).

Anti-aging

Hemp CBD is a powerful antioxidant[4] (A.J. Hampson et al). Antioxidants play an important role in protecting the skin from free radicals, such as UV rays, smoke, and environmental pollutants. In the anti-aging market, the value of hemp CBD as an antioxidant is exceptionally promising since fine lines and wrinkles are caused by free radicals, which accelerate the aging process and decreases skin elasticity. There is no question about Hemp CBD being a powerful antioxidant. The US government's patent confirms cannabinoids as both a neuroprotectant and antioxidant. From the patent 1999/008769, "cannabinoids have been found to have antioxidant properties...makes cannabinoids useful in the treatment and prophylaxis of a wide variety of oxidation associated diseases..."[5] An important definition to understand is prophylaxis, which means action taken to prevent disease.

Dr. Jeanette Jacknin said at the American Academy of Dermatology (AAD), "There are two recent studies that show the importance of CB1 receptors [cannabinoid receptor] in the skin for healthy basal cell regeneration. Basal cells have to regenerate and grow. If they don't, you look much older"[6] (Whitney Akers 2018).

Acne

The potential for acne products using hemp CBD is huge. Not only because it is a highly effective anti-inflammatory, but also because it is highly effective at reducing the amount of sebum, or skin oils, produced by the body[7] (Nóra Dobrosi et al 2008). This is incredibly promising for the production of natural acne products, rather than those which use the common and harsh chemical agents such as benzoyl peroxide or a retinoid.

The three major causes of acne are sebum over-production, overactive sebocytes (cells of the sebaceous glands), and inflammation. A 2014 study concluded that CBD plays a key role in the regulation of sebum production and reduces the proliferation of sebocytes[8] (Attila Oláh et al 2014). We've already established that hemp CBD reduces inflammation, which rounds out hemp CBD as a powerful ingredient in the anti-acne market. Since stress and hormone changes play such an important role in acne, the internal use of hemp CBD oil to help the endocannabinoid system can address acne from a variety of body systems.

The CBD treatment of allergies, acne, cancer, and so many other skin abnormalities are promising, since a 2013 study found that cannabinoids could help control cell proliferation and differentiation[9] (Galve-Roperh et al 2013).

Skin Issues Related to the Immune System

In addition, skincare issues related to an imbalance in the immune system, such as eczema and psoriasis, can be treated with hemp CBD. The support hemp CBD gives to the immune system can help from the inside out and outside in with the use of both topical and internal products. There is significant data demonstrating that CB2 receptors have been found on immune cells, suggesting that cannabinoids play an important role in the regulation of the immune system[10] (G.A. Cabral and L. Griffin-Thomas 2009). Many skin conditions are a reaction of the immune system.

A 2015 study demonstrated that a molecule interacting with the endocannabinoid system inhibited mast cell activation[11] (Valerio Chiurchiu et al 2015). Mast cells are immune cells that release histamine when activated, which leads to intense itching and inflammation. This could have massive implications for those suffering with the currently incurable mast cell activation syndrome and overall for those suffering from allergic reactions.

Since psoriasis is an inflammatory disease that is characterized by the hyper-proliferation of the epidermal keratinocyte, it has been hard to treat, and nearly impossible to address naturally. However, since keratinocytes have a functional endocannabinoid system, hemp CBD has a promising future in the treatment of psoriasis. A 2007 study found that cannabinoids inhibit keratinocyte proliferation, and therefore supports a potential role for cannabinoids in the treatment of psoriasis[12] (Wilkinson JD and Williamson EM 2007).

As an aromatherapist and cosmetic formulator, one of the most common requests for a topical product is one to address eczema. The eczema rash is a symptom of a bigger problem. I could help with the pain and appearance of eczema, but I could not address the underlying immune response. There is promising potential for relief with internal and external use of hemp CBD, along with a careful study of what environmental elements or foods are contributing to the exaggerated immune response.

In the United States 31.6 million Americans are affected by eczema including infants, children and adults[13] (National Eczema Association). The cycle of eczema is hard to break. With eczema, an overactive immune system causes the skin to break out in rashes. A University of Colorado School of Medicine study found that 8 out of the 21 patients that applied cannabinoid creams twice a day for three weeks noticed a significant improvement in their severely itchy skin. Dr. Robert Dellavalle said, "Perhaps the most promising role for cannabinoids is in the treatment of itch"[14] (Science News 2017). According to an article from the National Eczema Association, "with measurable anti-itch, anti-pain, anti-microbial and anti-inflammatory properties, the effect of cannabinoids in patients with atopic dermatitis [eczema] has already begun to be demonstrated"[15] (Peter Lio, M.D. et al 2017).

Cancer

A 2013 study found that cannabinoids possess anti-proliferative and pro-apoptotic effects, and they are known to interfere with tumour neovascularization, cancer cell migration, adhesion, invasion, and metastasization. Advancement in cannabinoid use in cancer treatment came from the discovery of a potential use of cannabinoids in targeting and killing cancer cells[16] (Paola Massi et al).

Hemp CBD shows promise in the study of skin cancer. An article in the Journal of Dermatology and Clinical Research found, "An assessment of the available findings indicates that components of the endocannabinoid system (ECS) play an important role in the development of Non-Melanoma Skin Cancer (NMSC) and melanoma which have a higher incidence than all other cancers combined. The ECS is involved in the formation of UVB-induced NMSC and melanoma. Endocannabinoids, synthetic cannabinoids and phytocannabinoids decrease NMSC and melanoma growth in vitro and in vivo through CB receptor dependent and independent pathways. This suggests that molecules which make up the ECS are potential targets for development of novel skin cancer therapeutics. Because NMSC and melanoma rates are rapidly increasing, new therapeutic options are needed"[17] (Soliman E. et al 2016).

Pain

The authors of "Non-psychotropic plant cannabinoids: new therapeutic opportunities from an ancient herb" wrote, "More recently, CBD was shown to be effective in well-established experimental models of analgesia, as well as in acute and chronic models of inflammation in rodents. It is believed that the analgesic effect of CBD is mediated, at least in part, by TRPV1 and that its anti-arthritic action is due to a combination of immunosuppressive and anti-inflammatory effects"[18] (Angelo A. Izzo et al 2009).

It is believed that hemp CBD works faster for localized issues when used topically because the CBD goes directly to the CB1 and CB2 cannabinoid receptor sites in the specific area that it is applied, without going through the digestive system. In a study, transdermal CBD significantly reduced joint swelling, improved mobility, and reduced pain for rats with arthritis[19] (D.C. Hammell et al 2016).

Topicals are applied right to trouble areas so that the CBD oil can work directly where it's needed most. Ingesting CBD products orally causes CBD and other compounds to enter the blood stream, which elicits full-body effects and takes up to 2 hours or more before those effects are experienced. With CBD topicals, the healing compound and other hemp-derived nutrients are almost immediately absorbed directly through your skin, allowing them to target the affected area for quicker and more focused effects. The analgesic, anti-inflammatory, and neuroprotective effects of hemp CBD work together for some impressive and sometimes shocking pain relief.

Chapter 5
The Business of Hemp CBD in Skincare

So here is the rub—now that you know the incredible healing properties of hemp CBD—you cannot use any of it to sell and promote hemp CBD. As both consumers and business owners, it is vital to understand the rules and regulations that govern the topical application and internal use of hemp CBD.

Among other things, the FDA is in charge of food, cosmetics, and drugs. As a topical product, hemp CBD products fall under the purview of cosmetics with the FDA. There is a fine line between drugs and cosmetics. It is important that we clearly stay on our side of the line, and not walk the tightrope between the two definitions.

Let's talk first about the role the FDA plays in cosmetics. The FDA has authority over cosmetics. The *intended use* of a cosmetic determines whether it falls under a cosmetic or a drug. Claims that are made on the packaging, on social media, websites, consumer reviews, or any advertising that can sway what the consumer believes the product will do, can change what the FDA views as the intended use of a product.

To navigate the concept of intended use, it is vital to know how the FDA defines a cosmetic and a drug. According to the Federal Food, Drug, and Cosmetic Act (FD&C Act) cosmetics are "articles intended to be rubbed, poured, sprinkled, or sprayed on, introduced into, or otherwise applied to the human body or any part thereof for cleansing, beautifying, promoting attractiveness, or altering the appearance" (FD&C Act, sec. 201(i)).

When it comes to drugs, a cosmetic can become a drug if claims make the intended use "for therapeutic use, such as treating or preventing disease, or to affect the structure or function of the body." Cosmetics have simple labeling regulations and voluntary adverse effects reporting. You cannot make any claims other than cosmetic usage, even if it is accurate or nature's wonder "drug."

The manufacturer is responsible for making cosmetics safe, and they must not be adulterated or misbranded. Adulterated is defined as harmful or injurious to users under customary conditions of use, such as microbiology, unapproved color additive, chemical contaminant, or prohibited ingredient. And misbranded is defined as when labeling is false or misleading; package does not exhibit labeling information required by statute or regulation; packaging not in compliance with 1970 Poison Prevention Packaging Act (PPPA); or the packaging lacks required information.

All cosmetic ingredient lists are required to use INCI (International Nomenclature of Cosmetic Ingredients) names for all cosmetic ingredients in a finished product, and they must be listed in descending order. The use of trade or common names is not allowed on cosmetic ingredient lists.

There are some that claim, "If you can't pronounce it, it can't be good for you." This statement was made by the Environmental Working Group and placed on a banner at Natural Products Expo. It should take the award as the most uninformed, illogical statement ever made by a political action group.

International standardization to ensure consumer safety worldwide means that we can't just put everything into basic English. It means that some words in cosmetic labeling will be difficult to pronounce; I still can't say *Butyrospermum parkii*, but Shea Butter is as safe as ingredients come. Whether you can pronounce the INCI term or not, the use of INCI nomenclature is the law.

Let me reiterate that the all cosmetic ingredients must be listed on the label in *descending order*. I have seen countless bath bombs and topical products that list hemp CBD as the very first ingredient. We all know that we'd have to be selling our products for insane amounts if hemp CBD was the very first ingredient. It has to be dissolved or carried in some sort of ingredient first, which often it isn't even making the list! Also every single bath bomb on the face of the earth is predominantly made with baking soda and citric acid. *How can hemp CBD possibly be the very first ingredient?* It can't. It is physically impossible.

Speaking of labels, the FDA does regulate what must be on the label of your product. These include: an identity statement, an accurate statement of the net quantity of contents, name and place of business, distributor statement, material facts, warning and caution statements, and ingredients. FDA labeling requirements can be found on the FDA website, but if you really want to understand labeling, I highly recommend Marie Gale's book, *Soap & Cosmetic Labeling: How to Follow the Rules and Regs Explained in Plain English.*

So why be a cosmetic over a drug?

Cosmetics do not require pre-market clearance, or approval by the FDA, and registration with the FDA is currently voluntary. The FDA suggests that a brand can reduce the risk of adulterated or misbranded cosmetics if you manufacture following current GMP, however it does not require that they are followed.

On the other hand, drugs are highly regulated and require pre-clearance by the FDA, and cGMP is required. Drugs have highly regulated labeling laws (i.e. Drug Facts). They require reporting of all and any adverse effects known, and they can make proven, specific, and tested claims that follow the monographs requirements.

In the Drug Legality Principle, a product meets the definition of a drug if it complies with ALL requirements for drugs (even if it also meets the definition of a cosmetic). A product is considered a drug if it makes claims such as being a sunscreen, antibacterial soap, anti-dandruff shampoo, anti-acne, anti-wrinkle, antiperspirant, etc.

While your hemp CBD product may be the be-all and end-all of natural cures, you simply cannot make that claim because your intended use claims will convert your hemp CBD cosmetic product into a drug.

Three Types of Claims that Make Your Cosmetic a Drug

1. Claims that suggest physiological change. For instance, if you say, "younger looking" rather than "younger" you are a cosmetic. If you say "removes" or "prevents" wrinkles, rather than "covers" your product is a drug.
2. Claims that sound scientific. For instance, if you claim that your soaps are "Compounded in our laboratory under the most sterile conditions" or "If blemishes persist, see a doctor," your products is a drug.
3. Claims that appear in an applicable OTC monograph, such as sunscreen products, hormone products, acne, eczema, psoriasis, skin bleaching, etc. Even implied claims by known effects of ingredients.

The trick is this: it doesn't matter whether the claim is true or not, it's whether the claim transforms the cosmetic into a drug.

A few marketing ploys that can get you in trouble with the FDA, and alert knowledgeable consumers that you don't know the laws of the industry you're in, include:

- making claims your product is FDA approved.
- or that your facility is an FDA approved facility.
- making product claims based on known effects of ingredients.
- unsubstantiated endorsements (such as Celebrity Infomercials) or product reviews.
- a disclaimer such as "results may vary" or "not typical for the average consumer."
- The use of the term "cosmeceuticals" for your product is a big red flag because a product can be a drug, cosmetic, or a combination of both, following the rules of both standards. But the term "cosmeceutical" has no meaning under the law.

Your Product's Intended Use Can Make Your Cosmetic a Drug

Example #1: Product's Intended Use: Drug—A product with any of the following intended uses is a drug: antiperspirant/deodorant (stops perspiration), dandruff shampoo (treats dandruff), sunscreen/suntan preparation (prevents sunburn), fluoride toothpaste (prevents cavities), and skin protectant (helps heal cuts).

Example #2: Product's Intended Use: Cosmetic—A product with any of the following intended uses is a cosmetic: deodorant (covers up odor), shampoo (cleanses hair), suntan preparation (moisturizes while tanning), toothpaste (cleans teeth or freshens breath), skin protectant (moisturizes skin). Notice that both the ingredients and the intended use of the product make a difference in whether it is considered a drug or a cosmetic.

But Other Companies Do It

Just because you see another company making claims does not mean you should. If the FDA looks into your claim, you can't use another company's bad judgment as an excuse for your choices. Claims can put a company into the drug side of the FDA, which would make them out of compliance. As a cosmetic formulator who has worked on OTC sunscreen products, I would rue the day that hemp CBD becomes an over-the-counter drug. The cost, paperwork, and red tape of hemp CBD becoming an OTC drug would put 99.9% of small businesses out of business.

Good Manufacturing Practices and You

Current Good Manufacturing Practice (GMP) guidelines are important for any size business to be familiar with. When proper cleanliness is not maintained, your product can be deemed adulterated or misbranded, and you will be prohibited from selling it.

Following GMP is not required for cosmetic products, but the practices are worth knowing and working towards. No matter how much product you sell or how small your company is, now is a good time to implement as many GMP practices into your business as possible and to keep up with the revisions.

I recommend addressing GMP guidelines in bite-size chunks. How do you eat an elephant? That's right: one bite at a time. The entire GMP guidelines can be found on the FDA website at FDA.gov/CosmeticGuidances. While following cGMP is not currently the law, Congress has had one bill after another up for discussion for years. Something will eventually pass, and it is certain to include mandatory GMP.

About The Author

Kayla Fioravanti is a certified aromatherapist, award-winning author, cosmetic formulator, and hemp expert. In 1998 Kayla co-founded Essential Wholesale, which was listed as one of *INC Magazine's 5000 Fastest Growing Companies in America* three years in a row. Essential Wholesale began in Kayla's kitchen with a $50 investment in 1998, and sold for millions in 2011.

Kayla is a serial entrepreneur. After selling Essential Wholesale, she founded Selah Press, followed by the launch of Ology Essentials, a research-driven brand of high quality hemp products, fluffery-free aromatherapy certification program, experience-based business consulting, and honest no-hype custom formulating services. Ology Essentials is an indispensable aromatherapy and natural products resource and supplier. Kayla is an approved school educator by the National Association of Holistic Aromatherapists.

Kayla's writing is a sincere reflection of who she is. She writes everything from poetry to textbooks used in natural medicine programs. Kayla loves to research complex problems, dissect the information to its smallest component, and then write it for her readers in everyday English.

Kayla's books include: *The Unspoken Truth About Essential Oils* with Stacey Haluka; *The Art, Science and Business of Aromatherapy*; *DIY Kitchen Chemistry*; *How to Make Melt & Pour Soap Base from Scratch* along with 7 other books available on Amazon.

Kayla lives in Franklin, Tennessee with her family and a whole host of critters. She can be found at Ology Essentials working diligently on innovative formulations, supporting other small businesses as they enter the hemp CBD industry, and building a family based business with Keegan, Haleigh Fioravanti and the rest of the Ology Essentials team. You can reach her at kayla@ologyessentials.com or follow her blogs on OlogyEssentials.com and KaylaFioravanti.com.

References

Chapter 1

[1] World Health Organization. CANNABIDIOL (CBD) Pre-Review Report Agenda, Item 5.2 Expert Committee on Drug Dependence   6-10 November 2017. PDF.
http://www.who.int/medicines/access/controlled-substances/5.2_CBD.pdf

[2] Bergamaschi, Mateus Machado; Queiroz, Regina Helena Costa; Zuardi, Antonio Waldo; Crippa, Jose Alexandre. Safety and Side Effects of Cannabidiol, a Cannabis sativa Constituent. Current Drug Safety. 2011. WEB.
http://www.eurekaselect.com/75752/article

[3] Iffland, Kerstin and Grotenhermen, Franjo. Cannabis and Cannabinoid Research, Volume 2, No. 1. An Update on Safety and Side Effects of Cannabidiol: A Review of Clinical Data and Relevant Animal Studies. 2017. WEB. https://www.liebertpub.com/doi/full/10.1089/can.2016.0034

[4] Patent US6630507B1 US Grant, US Department of Health and Human Services (HHS). Google Patent. Cannabinoids as antioxidants and neuroprotectants. 1998. WEB.
https://patents.google.com/patent/US6630507B1/en

[5] Iffland, Kerstin and Grotenhermen, Franjo. Cannabis and Cannabinoid Research, Volume 2, No. 1. An Update on Safety and Side Effects of Cannabidiol: A Review of Clinical Data and Relevant Animal Studies. 2017. WEB. https://www.liebertpub.com/doi/full/10.1089/can.2016.0034

[6] Iffland, Kerstin and Grotenhermen, Franjo. Cannabis and Cannabinoid Research, Volume 2, No. 1. An Update on Safety and Side Effects of Cannabidiol: A Review of Clinical Data and Relevant Animal Studies. 2017. WEB. https://www.liebertpub.com/doi/full/10.1089/can.2016.0034

Chapter 2

[1] Ministry of Hemp. Hemp vs Marijuana; What Makes Hemp Different from Marijuana. Miji Media LLC. 2018. WEB.
https://ministryofhemp.com/hemp/not-marijuana/

[2] West, David Ph.D. North American Industrial Hemp Council. Hemp Myths and Realities. Ecomall. WEB.
https://www.ecomall.com/greenshopping/hempmyths.htm

[3] Leaf Science. 5 Differences Between Hemp and Marijuana. 2014. WEB.
https://www.leafscience.com/2014/09/16/5-differences-hemp-marijuana/

[4] Rothenberg, Erik. A RENEWAL OF COMMON SENSE, The Case for Hemp in 21st Century America. Vote Hemp, INC. 2001. WEB.
https://www.votehemp.com/wp-content/uploads/2018/09/renewal.pdf

[5] Jacknin, Jeanette. Cannabinoids in Hemp for Beauty, Skin Health. Natural Products Insider. 2016. WEB.
https://www.naturalproductsinsider.com/beauty/cannabinoids-hemp-beauty-skin-health

[6] Say No to Palm Oil. What's the Issue? 2018. WEB.
http://www.saynotopalmoil.com/Whats_the_issue.php

[7] MSMV News. News 4. Murfreesboro woman loses job after taking CBD. August 6, 2018. WEB. https://www.wsmv.com/news/murfreesboro-woman-loses-job-after-taking-cbd/video_b1bb68a3-5aab-5659-960b-575b53c17ba1.html

[8] Pappas, Robert PhD. Cannabis Confusion: Hemp, Marijuana, CBD, and THC. Essential Oil University Facebook Page. February 23, 2017. WEB.
https://www.facebook.com/note.php?note_id=10155147183928083

Chapter 3

[1] Dustin Sulak, D.O. The Endocannabinoid System. Healer. 2016. WEB.
https://healer.com/the-endocannabinoid-system/

[2] Rodolfo, Kevin. What is Homeostasis? Emeritus Professor Kelvin Rodolfo of the University of Illinois at Chicago's Department of Earth and Environmental Sciences provides this answer. WEB.
https://www.scientificamerican.com/article/what-is-homeostasis/

[3] Russo, E.B. Clinical endocannabinoid deficiency (CECD): can this concept explain therapeutic benefits of cannabis in migraine, fibromyalgia, irritable bowel syndrome, and other treatment-resistant conditions. PubMed. Us National Library of Medicine National Institute of Health. 2004. WEB.
https://www.ncbi.nlm.nih.gov/pubmed/15159679

[4] National Institute of Health. U.S. National Library of Medicine. National Center for Biotechnology Information. PubChem. Open Chemistry Data Base. Compound Summary for CID 644019, Cannabidiol. WEB. https://pubchem.ncbi.nlm.nih.gov/compound/cannabidiol#section=Top

Chapter 4

[1] Ständer S; Schmelz M; Metze D; Luger T; Rukwied R. Distribution of cannabinoid receptor 1 (CB1) and 2 (CB2) on sensory nerve fibers and adnexal structures in human skin. U.S. National Library of Medicine. National Institutes of Health. 2005. WEB. https://www.ncbi.nlm.nih.gov/pubmed/15927811

[2] Mauro Maccarrone; Marianna Di Rienzo; Natalia Battista; Valeria Gasperi; Pietro Guerrieri; Antonello Rossi; and Alessandro Finazzi-Agrò. The Endocannabinoid System in Human Keratinocytes. Evidence That Anandamide Inhibits Epidermal Differentiation Through CB1 Receptor-Dependent Inhibition Of Protein Kinase C, Activating Protein-1, And Transglutaminase. U.S. National Library of Medicine. National Institutes of Health. 2003. WEB. http://www.jbc.org/content/278/36/33896.full

[3] Tamás Bíró; Balázs I. Tóth; György Haskó; Ralf Paus; and Pál Pacher. The endocannabinoid system of the skin in health and disease: novel perspectives and therapeutic opportunities. U.S. National Library of Medicine. National Institutes of Health. 2009. WEB. https://www.ncbi.nlm.nih.gov/pmc/articles/PMC2757311/

[4] A. J. Hampson; M. Grimaldi; J. Axelrod; and D. Wink. Cannabidiol and (−)Δ9-tetrahydrocannabinol are neuroprotective antioxidants. U.S. National Library of Medicine. National Institutes of Health. 1998. WEB. https://www.ncbi.nlm.nih.gov/pmc/articles/PMC20965/

[5] Patent US6630507B1 US Grant, US Department of Health and Human Services (HHS). Google Patent. Cannabinoids as antioxidants and neuroprotectants. 1998. WEB. https://patents.google.com/patent/US6630507B1/en

[6] Akers, Whitney. Cannabis Could Be the New Super Ingredient in Skin Care. The potential for topical CBD treatments doesn't end with acne. They may also help people with psoriasis get relief with minimal side effects. Healthline. 2018. WEB. https://www.healthline.com/health-news/cannabis-the-new-super-ingredient-in-skin-care#1

[7] Nóra Dobrosi; Balázs I. Tóth; Georgina Nagy; Anikó Dózsa; Tamás Géczy;

László Nagy; Christos C. Zouboulis; Ralf Paus; László Kovács; and Tamás Bíró. Endocannabinoids enhance lipid synthesis and apoptosis of human sebocytes via cannabinoid receptor-2-mediated signaling. The FASEB Journal. 2008. WEB. https://www.fasebj.org/doi/abs/10.1096/fj.07-104877?sid=708a0456-85c6-48b8-b0b6-5e0ecdf64528

[8] Attila Oláh; Balázs I. Tóth; István Borbíró; Koji Sugawara; Attila G. Szöllõsi; Gabriella Czifra; Balázs Pál; Lídia Ambru; Jennifer Kloepper; Emanuela Camera; Matteo Ludovici; Mauro Picardo; Thomas Voets; Christos C. Zouboulis; Ralf Paus; and Tamás Bíró. Cannabidiol exerts sebostatic and anti-inflammatory effects on human sebocytes. U.S. National Library of Medicine. National Institutes of Health. 2014. WEB. https://www.ncbi.nlm.nih.gov/pmc/articles/PMC4151231/

[9] Galve-Roperh; Chiurchiù V'; Díaz-Alonso J; Bari M; Guzmán M; and Maccarrone M. Cannabinoid receptor signaling in progenitor/stem cell proliferation and differentiation. U.S. National Library of Medicine. National Institutes of Health. 2013. WEB. https://www.ncbi.nlm.nih.gov/pubmed/24076098

[10] G.A. Cabral and L. Griffin-Thomas. Emerging Role of the CB2 Cannabinoid Receptor in Immune Regulation and Therapeutic Prospects. U.S. National Library of Medicine. National Institutes of Health. 2009. WEB. https://www.ncbi.nlm.nih.gov/pmc/articles/PMC2768535/

[11] Valerio Chiurchiù; Luca Battistini; and Mauro Maccarrone. Endocannabinoid signaling in innate and adaptive immunity. U.S. National Library of Medicine. National Institutes of Health. 2015. WEB. https://www.ncbi.nlm.nih.gov/pmc/articles/PMC4557672/

[12] Wilkinson JD and Williamson EM. Cannabinoids inhibit human keratinocyte proliferation through a non-CB1/CB2 mechanism and have a potential therapeutic value in the treatment of psoriasis. U.S. National Library of Medicine. National Institutes of Health. 2007. WEB. https://www.ncbi.nlm.nih.gov/pubmed/17157480

[13] National Eczema Association. Eczema Facts. WEB. https://nationaleczema.org/research/eczema-facts/

[14] Science News. Cannabinoids may soothe certain skin diseases, say researchers. Anti-inflammatory properties may be the key. 2017. WEB. https://www.sciencedaily.com/releases/2017/04/170418094315.htm

[15] Peter Lio, M.D.; Helena Yardley, Ph.D. Franklin BioScience; and Jon Fernandez, SVP Franklin BioScience. Can marijuana help eczema? A medical doctor and researchers in the cannabis industry explain the science behind cannabis as a potential treatment for atopic dermatitis. National Eczema Association. 2017. WEB. https://nationaleczema.org/can-marijuana-help/

[16] Paola Massi; Marta Solinas; Valentina Cinquina; and Daniela Parolaro. Cannabidiol as potential anti-cancer drug. U.S. National Library of Medicine. National Institutes of Health. 2013. WEB. https://www.ncbi.nlm.nih.gov/pmc/articles/PMC3579246/

[17] Soliman E.; Ladin DA; and Rukiyah Van Dross. Cannabinoids as Therapeutics for Non-Melanoma and Melanoma Skin Cancer. SciMedCentral. Journal of Dermatology and Clinical Research. 2016. WEB. https://www.jscimedcentral.com/Dermatology/dermatology-4-1069.pdf

[18] Angelo A. Izzo; Francesca Borrelli; Raffaele Capasso; Vincenzo Di Marzo; and Raphael Mechoulam. Non-psychotropic plant cannabinoids: new therapeutic opportunities from an ancient herb. Cell Press. 2009. WEB. http://www.stcm.ch/en/files/paper_izzo_tips_2009.pdf

[19] D.C. Hammell; L.P. Zhang; F. Ma; S.M. Abshire; S.L. McIlwrath; A.L. Stinchcomb; and K.N. Westlund. Transdermal cannabidiol reduces inflammation and pain-related behaviours in a rat model of arthritis. U.S. National Library of Medicine. National Institutes of Health. 2016. WEB. https://www.ncbi.nlm.nih.gov/pmc/articles/PMC4851925/

Chapter 5

FDA Code of Regulations. *CFR-Code of Federal Regulations Title 21*. U.S. Food and Drug Administration. April 1, 2017. Retrieved from https://www.accessdata.fda.gov/scripts/cdrh/cfdocs/cfCFR/CFRSearch.cfm?fr=201.303

FDA, U.S. Food and Drug Administration. *Cosmetics,* http://www.fda.gov/Cosmetics/default.htm

FDA, U.S. Food and Drug Administration. *Cosmetics Labeling and Label Claims,* http://www.fda.gov/Cosmetics/CosmeticLabelingLabelClaims/default. htm

FDA, U.S. Food and Drug Administration. *Federal Food, Drug, and Cosmetics Act (FD and C Act),* http://www.fda.gov/RegulatoryInformation/Legislation/FederalFoodDruga

ndCosmeticActFDCAct/default.htm

FDA, U.S. Food and Drug Administration. *Good Manufacturing Practice (GMP) Guildelines/Inspections Checklist,*
http://www.
fda.gov/Cosmetics/GuidanceComplianceRegulatoryInformation/
GoodManufacturingPracticeGMPGuidelinesInspectionChecklist/default.htm

FDA, U.S. Food and Drug Administration. *Guidance, Compliance and Regulatory Information,*
http://www.fda.gov/Cosmetics/GuidanceComplianceRegulatoryInformation
/default.htm

FDA, U.S. Food and Drug Administration. *Is It a Cosmetic, a Drug, or Both? (Or Is It Soap?),*
http://www.fda.gov/Cosmetics/GuidanceComplianceRegulatoryInformation
/ucm074201.htm

FDA, U.S. Food and Drug Administration. *Product and Ingredient Safety,*
http://www.fda.gov/Cosmetics/ProductandIngredientSafety/default.htm